Women's Health

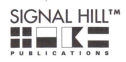

SIGNAL HILL™

PUBLICATIONS

Copyright © 1997
Signal Hill Publications
An imprint of New Readers Press
U.S. Publishing Division of Laubach Literacy International
Box 131, Syracuse, New York 13210-0131

Information graphics by Fran Forstadt
Illustrations by Linda Alden
Cover photo: P. Beaurline/SUPERSTOCK
Cover design: Kimbrly Koennecke

9 8 7 6 5 4 3 2 1

Library of Congress Cataloging-in-Publication Data

Women's health.
p. cm. — (For your information)
ISBN 1-56853-034-X (pbk.)
1. Women—Health and hygiene. 2. Women's health services. I. Series: FYI (Syracuse, N.Y.)
RA778.W7532   1997
613'.04244—dc21   96-50012
                                    CIP

Contents

Preface

Women have their own health care needs. To be healthy and live long, you need to know what those needs are. This book offers ideas about how to stay healthy and advice on dealing with health problems.

This book also gives information you need to seek help and get answers to your questions. It will help you be an active player in working with your doctor or other care providers.

Women's Health covers topics that affect only women, such as breast health. It also covers topics that affect women in different ways from men, such as aging. Health issues that affect both women and men similarly, such as skin cancer, are not covered in this book.

Some topics are not covered in detail. For example, pregnancy is covered only as it relates to other topics. This book is just a start to thinking about your health as a woman. Other sources include

- other women
- health care providers (doctors and nurses)

- support groups
- libraries

Women's Health was developed with Mary J. Breen, B.Sc., M.Ed. Ms. Breen is the author of *Taking Care: A Handbook about Women's Health.*

Thanks to the following people for their contribution to the content of *Women's Health:* Michele M. Sedor, Health Coordinator, The Literacy Project, Greenfield, MA; Diana North and Donna Swain, The North Quabbin Adult Education Center, MA; Donnica L. Moore, M.D.; Toni Cordell, New Reader Leadership Coordinator, Laubach Literacy; and the Reverend Senitila McKinley, member, Laubach Literacy Action Steering Committee.

Thanks to Susan James for research and to Jeanna Walsh for research and writing.

In this book

- *Care provider* refers to a doctor, nurse practitioner, family practice physician, or other licensed health care worker you see.

Chapter 1

Food

Eating healthy food has many benefits. Here are just a few:

- You feel better and have more energy.
- You are less likely to get sick.
- You can reach and stay at a healthy weight.
- You can reduce your risk of heart disease and stroke.
- You can reduce your risk of getting osteoporosis. (This is a disease that weakens your bones.)

Healthy Eating for Women

You can use the Food Guide Pyramid on page 11 to make healthy food choices. These guidelines will also help you:

- Eat many types of foods every day. This will help you get all the useful materials (nutrients) you need from food.
- Stay at a healthy weight. Being either too fat or too thin can harm your health. The chart below gives suggested healthy weight ranges for women.

Height (ft/ins)	Small frame	Medium frame	Large frame
4' 9"	99 – 108	106 – 118	115 – 128
4' 10"	100 – 110	108 – 120	117 – 131
4' 11"	101 – 112	110 – 123	119 – 134
5' 0"	103 – 115	112 – 126	121 – 137
5' 1"	105 – 118	115 – 129	125 – 140
5' 2"	108 – 121	118 – 132	128 – 144
5' 3"	111 – 124	121 – 135	131 – 148
5' 4"	114 – 127	124 – 138	134 – 152
5' 5"	117 – 130	127 – 141	137 – 156
5' 6"	120 – 133	130 – 144	140 – 160
5' 7"	123 – 136	133 – 147	143 – 164
5' 8"	126 – 139	136 – 150	146 – 167
5' 9"	129 – 142	139 – 153	149 – 170
5' 10"	132 – 145	142 – 156	152 – 173
5' 11"	135 – 148	145 – 159	155 – 176

Source: American Medical Association

- Choose a diet low in fat and cholesterol. This can reduce your risk of getting heart disease and some types of cancer. Many experts say that fat should make up no more than 30 percent of the calories you eat.

- Eat plenty of vegetables, fruits, and grains. These foods are usually low in fat and rich in nutrients. Grains include breads, cereals, pasta, and rice.

- Limit sugar in your diet. Foods high in sugar have calories, but few nutrients. Corn syrup, fructose, maltose, and lactose are all sugars.

- Limit salt in your diet. Salt contains sodium, and too much sodium increases your risk of having high blood pressure. Try using less table salt, and check the ingredients list on foods. Any ingredient that has *sodium, salt,* or *soda* as part of its name contains sodium.

- Limit alcohol in your diet. It has few nutrients and is linked with many health problems. If you are pregnant or trying to get pregnant, don't drink alcohol at all.

A note on convenience foods

Many prepared foods and "fast foods" do not help you eat healthfully. They often have a lot of sugar or sodium. They may be high in fat and calories, without providing nutrients.

It's always best to choose fresh foods.

For example, an orange soda is full of sugar and has few nutrients. But an orange or a glass of orange juice is packed with nutrients. Potato chips are made from potatoes, but they also contain a lot of salt and fat. A baked potato is a better choice.

The Food Guide Pyramid

The Food Guide Pyramid on page 11 shows you how much you should have each day from each food group. You should eat the *most* from the base of the pyramid and the least from the top. Try to stick as closely to the guidelines as you can.

Food Guide Pyramid

A guide to daily food choices

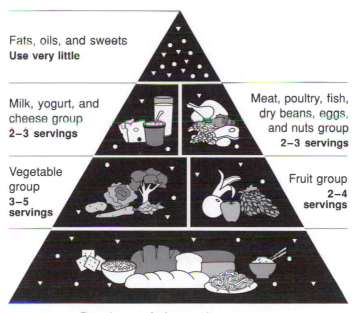

Fats, oils, and sweets
Use very little

Milk, yogurt, and cheese group
2–3 servings

Meat, poultry, fish, dry beans, eggs, and nuts group
2–3 servings

Vegetable group
3–5 servings

Fruit group
2–4 servings

Bread, cereal, rice, and pasta group
6–11 servings

Iron

Women need more iron than men do. When you have your period, you lose iron every month. To make up for this, you need to get iron from your food. Too little iron can cause anemia. Signs of anemia are tiredness, paleness, headaches, and getting sick often.

The best way to get enough iron is by eating the right foods. Good sources of iron are

- red meat and fish
- peas and beans
- spinach
- dried fruit
- whole grain products
- tofu

Your doctor may prescribe iron supplements. A supplement provides extra iron, usually in a pill.

Calcium

Women need more calcium than men do. Women have a higher risk of osteoporosis. Osteoporosis makes bones weak, so they break more easily.

Calcium helps to build bones. Getting enough calcium between the teenage years and age 35 is key. This is when the bones grow most. Up to age 24, women and girls need 1,200 milligrams (mg) of calcium a day. After that, women need 800 mg a day. If you are pregnant or breast-feeding, you need more.

Osteoporosis is most likely to happen after menopause. Experts suggest you get 1,500 mg of calcium a day. Most women need a calcium supplement after menopause.

The chart below lists some foods that are good sources of calcium.

Calcium in some foods

Food	Mg Calcium
broccoli, 1 cup, cooked	130
canned salmon with bones, 3 oz.	150
canned sardines with bones, 3 oz.	300
cheese, $1\frac{1}{2}$ oz.	300
cottage cheese, $\frac{1}{2}$ cup	75
dry beans, 1 cup, cooked	130
ice cream or frozen yogurt low fat, $\frac{1}{2}$ cup	100
milk, skim or low fat, 1 cup	300
tofu made with calcium, 4 oz.	120
yogurt, low fat or nonfat, 1 cup	350

Weight Control

Being overweight has some health risks, but dieting can also cause health problems. Many people are "yo-yo" dieters. They lose weight and then gain it back again and again. They are never able to keep the weight off.

Crash diets and diet pills may work, but only for a short time. You may lose a lot of weight quickly, but you will probably gain it back.

Yo-yo dieting puts a lot of strain on your heart. It also makes losing weight harder after every diet. If you crash diet for a long time, you may endanger your health.

> The best way to lose weight is to change what you eat and to exercise regularly.

Chapter 2, page 17, is about exercise and fitness. Talk to your care provider before you go on any diet or start an exercise program.

Losing weight safely

Here are some ideas for changing your eating habits:

- Forget about losing weight quickly. It took years to put on those extra pounds. It will take time to get rid of them.
- Keep a food diary for a week. Record
  — the amount
  — when and where you ate
  — why you ate. Were you hungry, or were you just bored?

  It may surprise you to see what you eat.

- Think about when and why you eat other than at mealtimes.
- Exercise. This will increase the number of calories your body uses. It will also build muscle. The more muscle you have, the better your body uses calories.
- Begin to change your unhealthy habits slowly. Start with small changes, one at a time.
- Let your body tell you when it needs food. Do not eat unless you are hungry.
- Do not forbid yourself certain foods. This will just make you want them more. If your favorite foods are high in fat or calories, eat them less often and in smaller amounts.

Getting help

Some people can't lose weight on their own. They need the help of a care provider or support group. Programs like Weight Watchers and Overeaters Anonymous can help, but be careful. Some programs cost a lot, and you may have to buy your food from them. Before you join, look into a few programs and talk to people who've tried them.

Eating Disorders

Some girls and women start dieting and cannot stop. They see themselves as fat, no matter how thin they get. They eat little or almost no food. These people have the eating disorder called anorexia.

Bulimia is another eating disorder. People with bulimia binge on food. They eat huge amounts. Then they vomit or use laxatives so they don't gain weight.

Eating disorders are very dangerous. Some girls and women starve themselves to death. Others harm their health forever. Anyone with an eating disorder needs to see a health care provider right away.

If you think someone you know has anorexia or bulimia, talk to her. Urge her to seek help. She can talk to her care provider. There are also support groups that can help. Help her find as much information as you can.

Chapter 2
Exercise

Regular exercise is one of the best things you can do for yourself. This is true for a woman at any age. Exercise can help you feel and look better. It can also make you healthier.

Exercise helps how you feel. Exercise

- reduces stress
- eases depression
- improves self-esteem
- gives you more energy

Exercise also helps your health in other ways. Exercise

- lowers blood pressure
- reduces risk of heart disease
- strengthens bones
- helps prevent osteoporosis
- helps you keep a healthy weight

How to Begin

Check with your care provider before starting to exercise. It's especially important to see a care provider first if you

- ❑ are over 40
- ❑ smoke
- ❑ have heart disease or a family history of heart disease
- ❑ have diabetes
- ❑ have dizzy spells
- ❑ have high cholesterol
- ❑ get out of breath after mild activity
- ❑ have bone or joint problems
- ❑ take medication

Be sure to check with your care provider if you have ever had chest pain while exercising.

Setting Your Goals

Look at the list below. Check the goals you would like to reach:

____ improve health

____ control weight

____ have more energy

____ improve how you look

____ improve flexibility

____ improve the way heart and lungs work

____ improve posture

____ lower cholesterol level

____ reduce depression or stress

____ make bones stronger

____ _____

____ _____

Add your own goals if they are different. Be sure your goals are within reach.

Choose an Activity and Stick with It

Here are some factors to think about when choosing the best activity for you:

- your goals and interests
- how much time you have
- your age and health
- the cost, if there is one

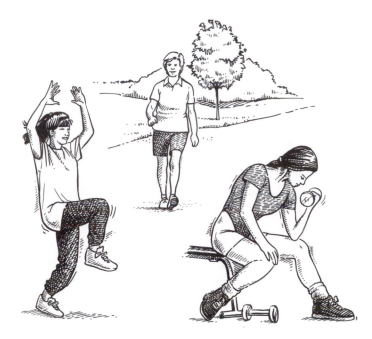

Possible activities include walking, running, jumping rope, biking, swimming, aerobics, basketball, and weight lifting.

☞ You should choose at least one activity that gets your heart beating faster.

Here are some tips about exercise:
- Don't expect to see results right away. It takes four to six weeks to notice real improvement.
- Set goals you can reach.

- Some exercise is better than no exercise.
- Buy good shoes that fit. Shoes that don't fit can cause painful feet or legs.
- Try exercising with a friend.

The Right Way

Whatever workout you choose should have three parts: the warm-up, the workout, and the cool-down.

Warm-up. Start your activity out slowly. You will reduce your risk of injuries if you warm up properly. Do a slow version of your main exercise, then stretch.

Workout. This is your main exercise, when you get your heart beating faster. Try to work out for 20 minutes, at least three times a week. As you exercise, you should be working hard, but not too hard.

If you are too out-of-breath to talk, you are probably working too hard.

Cool-down. When you finish, don't just stop. Instead, cool down for a few minutes. Do the same as your warm-up.

Everyday Exercise

Here are some ways to get a little bit of exercise every day:

- Walk whenever you can. When you take the car or bus, could you walk instead? If you take the bus, get off one stop earlier and walk the rest of the way. Take the stairs instead of the elevator.
- Think of household tasks as mini-workouts. Sweep or rake a little faster.
- Stretch or exercise while you watch TV.
- Stretch whenever you get the chance—at work or at home.

Osteoporosis and Exercise

Regular exercise reduces your risk of osteoporosis. Osteoporosis is a disease that weakens bones. It makes them break more easily.

To prevent bone loss as you get older, you need to exercise. The best exercises are the ones where you have to support your own weight. Be sure to include one or more of these in your fitness program:

- walking
- running
- lifting weights
- aerobics

Weight Control and Exercise

The best reasons to exercise are to feel better and be more healthy. Exercise can also help you lose weight. Regular exercise, combined with a healthy diet, is the best way to lose weight. Chapter 1, page 7, includes information about healthy eating.

Chapter 3

Smoking, Alcohol, and Drugs

Smoking and abusing alcohol or drugs can shorten your life. Cigarettes, alcohol, and drugs often affect women more strongly than men.

Smoking

Quitting smoking can add years to your life. On average, nonsmokers live five to eight years longer than smokers. The illustration on page 25 shows the health risks of smoking. Being around people who are smoking can harm your health, too.

The Risks of Smoking

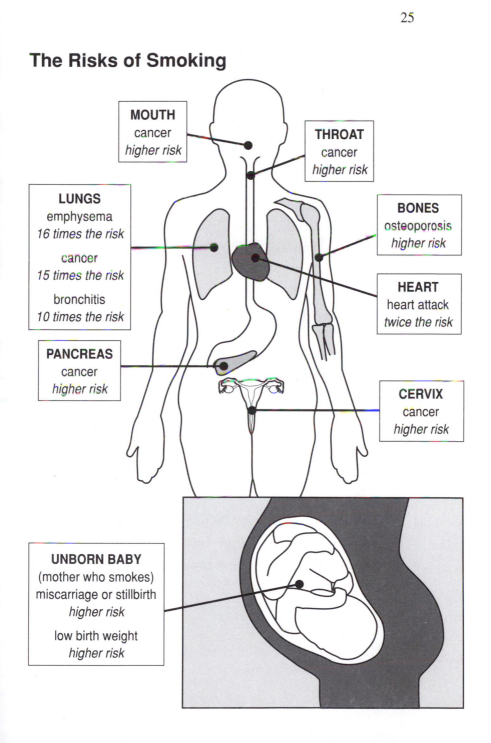

MOUTH
cancer
higher risk

THROAT
cancer
higher risk

LUNGS
emphysema
16 times the risk

cancer
15 times the risk

bronchitis
10 times the risk

BONES
osteoporosis
higher risk

HEART
heart attack
twice the risk

PANCREAS
cancer
higher risk

CERVIX
cancer
higher risk

UNBORN BABY
(mother who smokes)
miscarriage or stillbirth
higher risk

low birth weight
higher risk

┌──┐
│ Lung cancer is the number one cause of early deaths │
│ for women in the U.S.   │
└──┘

Most lung cancers are caused by smoking. Some are caused by being around other people's smoke.

Heart disease is also a major problem. Women who smoke and take birth control pills have a very high risk. They have 10 times the chance of getting heart disease that nonsmokers do. If you smoke *and* take birth control pills, talk to your care provider. She may suggest another form of birth control. Or she may get you help to quit smoking.

If you are pregnant, smoking can hurt your baby as well as you. Pregnant women who smoke are more likely to

- miscarry
- deliver a stillborn child
- deliver too early
- have a baby with low birth weight
- lose the baby to Sudden Infant Death Syndrome (SIDS). This is when babies die for no obvious cause.

Tips for quitting

⊘ Get rid of all cigarettes. Put away ashtrays, matches, and lighters.

⊘ Drink a lot of water. Try to stay away from coffee, alcohol, and sweets. They can make you want to smoke even more.

⊘ Get plenty of sleep and exercise. Eat healthy foods.

⊘ Keep your mouth and hands busy. Try chewing gum or sucking on a toothpick. Eat carrots or celery sticks. Play with a paper clip or squeeze a ball.

⊘ When you want a cigarette, take five slow, deep breaths.

⊘ Try a new exercise or hobby.

⊘ Tell your family and friends you are quitting. Ask them for help if you need it.

⊘ Think of yourself as a nonsmoker.

⊘ Be good to yourself. Many people "slip up." You haven't failed if you do. Just quit again.

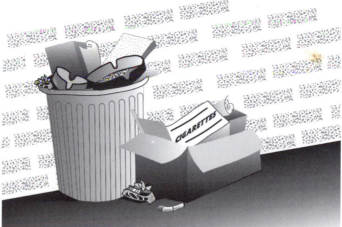

Quitting smoking

Quitting smoking is hard. It is also rewarding. More than 3 million people in the U.S. quit every year. When you quit, you can look forward to

- a lower risk of heart attack
- a lower risk of cancer
- feeling better

The tips on page 27 give ideas for quitting on your own. Some smokers need help to quit. Your doctor may prescribe nicotine gum or a nicotine patch. You can also buy gum and nicotine patches without a prescription. Check with your care provider, anyhow. Some people should not use these items. You can also join a self-help group. Page 94 lists places you can call for help.

Alcohol Abuse

Alcohol is the most abused drug in the U.S. Between 3 and 4 million women abuse alcohol. Here are the dangers for these women:

- They have a life span 15 years shorter than the average woman.
- They are more likely to be robbed, abused, or raped.

- They are more likely to be depressed.
- They have a higher risk of cancer.
- They have a higher risk of liver disease than men who abuse alcohol.
- They have a higher risk of damaging other organs, such as the heart.

Pregnant women who drink put their baby at risk. Alcohol use increases the chance of miscarriage and fetal alcohol syndrome. Fetal alcohol syndrome is the most common cause of mental retardation in babies.

Getting help for alcohol abuse

It may be hard to tell if you or someone you know has a drinking problem. Here are some warning signs to watch for:

- missing work because of a hangover
- blackouts
- fighting with family and friends because of alcohol
- not being able to do daily tasks because of alcohol
- drinking when alone
- drinking to calm down or ease stress
- having a drink first thing in the morning to get rid of a hangover

- being very drunk more than twice a year
- feeling guilty about drinking

If you have any of these warning signs, alcohol use is affecting your life. You need to seek help.

You can get help for an alcohol problem through treatment programs and self-help groups. You can find out about treatment programs from your care provider or a health clinic. Page 95 lists some other resources.

Drug Abuse

Using illegal drugs and using legal drugs in the wrong way are both drug abuse.

Some prescription drugs are addictive. They include tranquilizers, sleeping pills, amphetamines (stimulants), and painkillers.

It is dangerous to use more of these drugs than prescribed. Ignoring any of your care providers' instructions can be dangerous.

It's important to use *all* prescription drugs and over-the-counter drugs safely. Here are some tips:

- Ask your doctor about any drug she prescribes. Find out what it is for. Ask about side effects.

- Notice how any drug affects your body and your mind.
- Don't share prescription drugs with *anyone.*
- Never take a mood-altering drug within hours of using alcohol or another drug. Many drugs can have severe effects if taken together. Check with your care provider before taking any drugs at the same time.

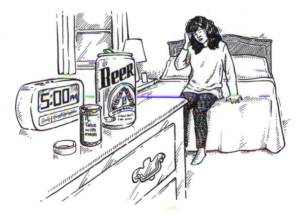

- Read any information that comes with the drug. Or ask the pharmacist to explain it.

Using illegal drugs can be dangerous. People who inject drugs may share needles. This increases their risk of getting hepatitis B and AIDS. Women who abuse drugs get sexually transmitted diseases (STDs) more often than other women. They may be trading sex for drugs, or they may have sex when their judgment is impaired by drugs.

If you are pregnant, cocaine and heroin can kill your baby or cause you to deliver early. Your baby can also be born addicted to these drugs.

Getting help for drug abuse

You can get help for drug abuse through treatment programs and self-help groups. You can find out about treatment programs from your care provider or a health clinic. Page 95 lists some resources for drug abuse problems.

Chapter 4

Doctor Visits

Staying healthy takes work. Women face many challenges in their work and family lives. It is important to take care of yourself and to have health care providers (doctors, nurses, and other health care workers) you can trust. They can help you stay healthy and prevent illness. They can also help you in emergencies.

There are many kinds of health care providers. All women should have a health care provider who does gynecological care. (This is care for a woman's reproductive system.) The chart below lists some care providers.

> **Obstetrician-gynecologists** are specialists. They have completed four or more years of training after medical school. They are trained in the field of women's reproductive health.
>
> **Internists** are specialists. They have three years of training beyond medical school. Some internists do gynecological exams.
>
> **Family doctors** have at least three years of general training after medical school. Doing gynecological exams is part of their practice. Some deliver babies.
>
> **Nurse practitioners** are registered nurses. They have extra training. They can perform some exams.
>
> **Nurse-midwives** are registered nurses. They have extra training and can deliver babies.

Primary Care Doctor

You may have more than one doctor. The most important is your primary care doctor. A primary care doctor may also be called an internist, a general practitioner (GP), or a family doctor. Some nurse practitioners do primary care. An obstetrician-gynecologist may be your primary care doctor if you are pregnant.

Your primary care doctor

- does routine checkups
- can treat many health problems
- is the one to call first if you are sick or hurt
- can send you to a specialist if you need one
- may perform pelvic exams and Pap tests (These are described on pages 37–39.)
- keeps your medical history on file

Clinics

If you don't have health insurance, you may not be able to afford a private doctor. A public health department clinic is a lower-cost option.

To find a clinic, call your county health or social services department. They can tell you about free or low-cost health clinics in your area.

If you get health care at a clinic, you may not see the same care provider each time. If this is the case, be sure each care provider you see knows your medical history.

Finding a Doctor

Don't wait until you are sick to find a doctor. You may need to try more than one doctor before you find the one that's right for you.

Here are some tips on finding a doctor:

- Ask family, friends, and coworkers.
- Check with the human resources office at your job.
- Ask another health care provider: a nurse, dentist, or pharmacist.
- Interview a new doctor. If you do not feel comfortable with him, find another doctor. Keep in mind that it takes time to build any relationship.

Some women prefer female care providers. They feel that women can understand their concerns more fully than men.

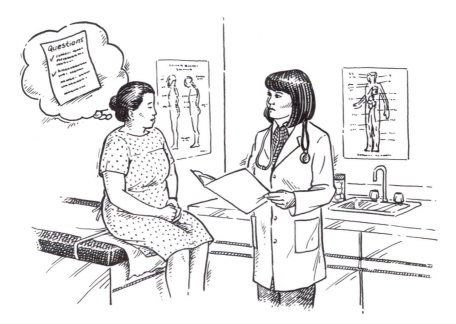

Routine Medical Exams

You and your care provider can work together. You can do some self-exams and watch for signs of problems. Your care provider can do medical exams and help you when there is a problem.

Once you choose a health care provider, you need to see him or her on a regular basis. Along with a medical checkup, he or she will suggest certain tests just for women. How often you have these tests depends on your age and medical history. The chart on page 38 tells who should have different medical tests.

Pelvic exam

During a pelvic exam your care provider looks at your outer sex organs. (Pages 57–58 describe a woman's outer sex organs.) She inserts a speculum into your vagina to let her see your cervix. The speculum holds the walls of your vagina apart.

Your care provider also examines your inner sex organs. She inserts two fingers into your vagina. With the other hand, she presses down on your stomach. This lets her feel the shape, size, and placement of your inner sex organs (see page 58). She may also perform a rectal exam.

Some Important Medical Tests for Women

Age 13–18	Age 19–39	Age 40–49	Age 50 and Older
■ Pap test and pelvic exam if sexually active ■ Pap test and pelvic exam starting at age 18 if not sexually active	■ pelvic exam every year ■ Pap test every year (after 3 normal tests in a row, patient and doctor may decide to do less often) ■ breast exam by a doctor every 3 years or more often ■ monthly BSE	■ pelvic exam every year ■ Pap test every year (after 3 normal tests in a row, patient and doctor may decide to do less often) ■ breast exam by a doctor every year ■ mammogram every 1–2 years* ■ monthly BSE	■ pelvic exam every year ■ Pap test every year (after 3 normal tests in a row, patient and doctor may decide to do less often) ■ breast exam by a doctor every year ■ mammogram every year ■ monthly BSE

* Many groups suggest you should start regular mammograms at age 40. They include the American Cancer Society and the National Cancer Institute. Other experts say you do not need regular mammograms before you are 50. If your family or medical history makes it more likely that you would get breast cancer, your doctor may start sooner.

Pap test

While the speculum is in, your care provider will take a small sample of cells from your cervix. This sample is sent to a lab to be tested. This is called a Pap test. It looks for early signs of cancer of the cervix.

Cancer of the cervix. Any woman can get cancer of the cervix. But some women are at higher risk of getting it. They include

- women who started having sex at an early age
- women who have had cancer of the cervix in the past
- women with many sexual partners
- women with a history of certain STDs (sexually transmitted diseases)
- women whose mothers took a drug called DES while they were pregnant
- women who smoke

Most cancers of the cervix can be either cured or prevented. Having a regular Pap test is key to preventing cancer of the cervix. The chart on page 38 shows who should have a Pap test and when.

If you have an abnormal Pap test, don't panic. Many abnormal cells are the result of other conditions, not cancer.

In some cases, treatment is needed. Most treatments involve medication. Other treatments remove the abnormal cells. Types of treatment include

- freezing the cells to remove them
- using a laser to remove the cells
- a cone biopsy (which removes large areas)

If you have cancer, treatment will be different. Your care provider may suggest surgery or radiation treatment. If your care provider suggests surgery, make sure it is needed. You may want to get a second opinion.

If the cancer has spread, your doctor may suggest chemotherapy. Ask questions about any treatment he suggests. Make sure you feel comfortable with the treatment. If you don't, you may need to seek a second opinion. The most major surgery would be hysterectomy—total removal of the uterus.

Breast exam

During an annual exam, your care provider will feel your breasts for lumps and other problems. She should also show you how to check your own breasts. This is called a breast self-exam (BSE). If she doesn't show you, ask her.

Women often find breast lumps by doing a breast self-exam. Doctors suggest that women over age 19 check their breasts every month. The best time to do a BSE is soon after your period ends. If you no longer have your period, you still need to do a BSE once a month. Choose a monthly date you can remember.

In a breast self-exam, you feel your breasts for lumps. You also feel for other changes. If you find any lumps or changes, ask your care provider to check them. Not every lump is cancer.

Page 43 shows a breast self-exam. Here's what to do:

1. Stand in front of a mirror. Look at your breasts. Are they the same as always? Check for dimples and scaly skin. Do your nipples leak? It's OK for your nipples to leak if you are pregnant or nursing. Otherwise, tell your care provider.

2. Put your hands behind your head. Press against your head. Do you see puckers or dimples now?

3. Put your hands on your hips. Pull your shoulders and elbows forward. Bend over a little. Do you see any puckers or dimples now?

Do steps 4 and 5 in the shower or lying
down. If you have large breasts, you should
probably do these steps lying down. This makes
it easier to feel the whole breast.

4. Lift your left arm over your head. Press
   the fingers of your right hand on your left
   breast. Begin at the outside edge. Move
   your fingers in small circles around the
   breast. Work toward the middle of the
   breast. Be sure to check the whole breast.
   Feel under the armpit, too. Feel for any
   lumps under the skin. Repeat with your
   left hand on your right breast.

5. Squeeze each nipple. Does anything come
   out?

If you notice any changes or lumps in your
breasts, see your care provider soon.

Mammogram

This is an X-ray of your breasts to check for
cancer. If you are over 40, your care provider
may suggest that you have regular mammograms.
Sometimes younger women need this test, too.

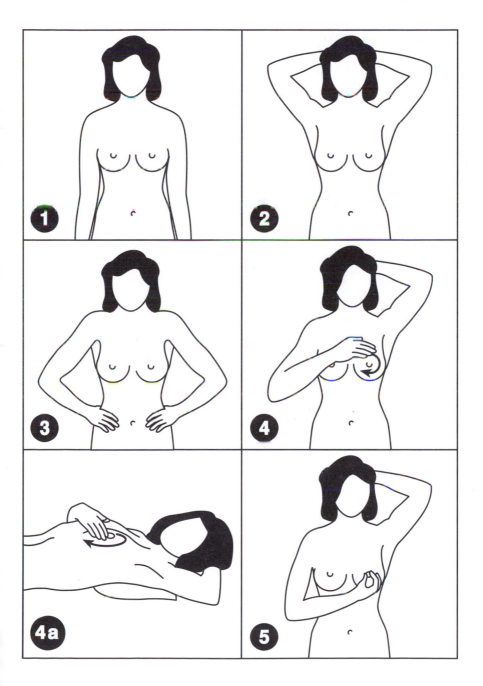

Breast Cancer

Breast cancer is the most common cancer in women. As many as 1 in every 8 women will get breast cancer in her lifetime.

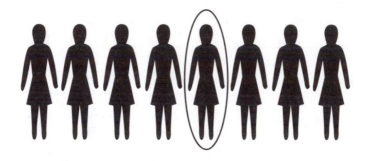

Some women are more likely than others to get breast cancer. They are

- women with a family history of breast cancer
- older women
- women who have never been pregnant
- women who have been pregnant only after age 30
- women who go through menopause late (still having periods at age 52)
- women whose periods started before they were 10
- women who regularly eat high-fat food

- women who have been exposed to radiation or certain chemicals
- women whose mothers took the drug DES when they were pregnant

This chapter has already described ways to check your breasts for signs of cancer. These checks are called breast cancer screening:

- breast self-exams
- exams by a care provider
- mammograms

These all look for early signs of cancer. The earlier cancer is found, the better your chances of successful treatment. Screening can save your life.

If you have signs of cancer, your care provider may do more tests. These can confirm if you have breast cancer. They could also rule it out if you don't. The tests could be

- another mammogram
- ultrasound (a test that uses sound waves to examine a breast lump)
- needle biopsy (A needle removes fluid from a breast lump. The fluid is tested for cancer.)
- biopsy (The lump is removed and tested. This is surgery.)

If your care provider wants to run more tests, find out why. Ask if you have options.

If you have breast cancer, the next step is treatment. This usually starts with removing the tumor. You may have either a lumpectomy or a mastectomy.

- A lumpectomy removes just the tumor. It may also remove some tissue around it.
- A mastectomy removes most or all of the breast.

After surgery, you may have radiation, chemotherapy, or both.

In most cases, you have a choice of the type of treatment. Talk to your doctor about your options. Get a second opinion if you are unsure.

Support groups

If you have breast cancer, a support group of other women who have it can be very helpful. It gives you a chance to find out about their experiences and how they cope. Ask your care provider how to find a group in your area.

Chapter 5

Mental Health Matters

The health of your body and mind are often linked. Today, we know that many illnesses are caused or made worse by stress. In fact, two out of every three visits to family doctors are for problems that may come from stress.

Stress can be especially hard on women. Many women work outside the home and have families to take care of. This can sometimes be too much to handle. Stress is the result.

Women are also more likely than men to suffer from depression. This chapter talks about both problems and gives some ideas for dealing with them.

Stress

You may feel stress when something good happens, or when something bad happens. You may also feel stress from your daily life. A little stress can help give you the energy to do what you need to do. But too much can harm you.

People with high stress levels are more likely to get sick. Important life events—good or bad—can cause a lot of stress. A death in the family or a divorce are high-stress events. So are getting married or retiring.

Signs of stress

Ongoing stress can lead to aches, pains, getting sick often, and sleep problems. At its worst, stress can lead to heart disease and ulcers. Some harmful signs of stress are

- tight muscles
- headaches, stomachaches, or backaches
- ulcers
- tiredness
- constipation or diarrhea
- fast heartbeat
- high blood pressure

- skin rashes
- urinating often
- weakness or dizziness
- depression
- crying easily
- bad temper
- eating, smoking, or drinking more

If you have any of the above symptoms, start by seeing your care provider. You may need help to reduce the stress in your life. A counselor can help with that.

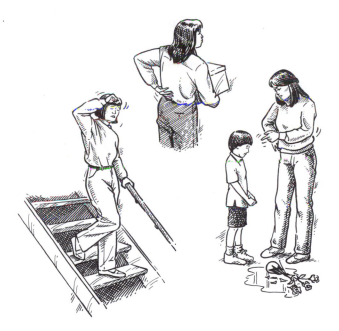

Handling stress

You need to find ways to stop stress from taking control of your life. Here are some tips for handling stress in your everyday life:

- Talk about your feelings or problems with someone you love.
- Get the sleep you need so that you're not tired during the day.
- Stay healthy: eat a balanced diet and exercise regularly.
- Take some time each day to relax. Take a walk or listen to music you like.
- Be a positive thinker. Reward yourself for what is going right before you worry about what may be wrong.
- Don't try to do many things at once. This may seem like a good way of getting things done, but it can make stress worse.
- Learn how to say "no." Realize that it's OK to say "no" when you can't do something (or just don't want to).

Counseling can also help. Your care provider can help you find a counselor.

Relaxing

Taking time to relax is a big part of reducing stress. Relaxing is a skill. It means "turning off" your mind for a while.

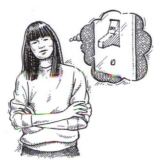

Here are some ways to relax. You can do them during the day when you start to feel stressed.

Deep breathing. Breathe from your stomach. Draw in a deep breath through your nose. Feel your lungs expand. Hold the breath for three seconds. Let the breath out slowly through your mouth. Keep doing this for three to five minutes.

Letting your mind wander. Set aside 15 minutes a day to clear your mind and let your thoughts wander. Do this in a quiet place. Close your eyes and try not to think of anything.

Relaxing your muscles. Try this exercise to release tension in your muscles. Sit or lie in a comfortable place. One at a time, tighten and relax all the different parts of your body. Start with your face and work down to your toes. Picture the stress leaving your body.

Stretching. Stand or lie down and stretch every part of you, as a cat does. Shake any areas that still feel tight. Move slowly and enjoy the way stretching feels.

Depression

Most people feel bad at some point in their lives. This feeling can last hours, or even days, and be normal. But when you feel bad for weeks or months at a time, you may have depression.

Depression is common. Millions of people suffer from it, and women are more likely to be depressed than men are. Depression can be treated with drugs, counseling, or both. Self-help groups can also help.

Short-term depression

Depression that lasts a few hours or days is short-term depression, or "the blues." Many things can cause short-term depression, such as

- problems in your relationships
- trouble at work

- your period
- hearing bad news
- the time of year (For example, a lot of people get depressed around the holidays.)

You can help yourself get over short-term depression. Talk to someone about how you feel. Try to stay busy. This can keep your mind off how you are feeling.

Exercise is another way to fight depression. Keeping active can help you feel more in control of your life.

You can also use some of the tips on page 50 for dealing with stress. Stress can often make you feel depressed for a while.

Long-term depression

Some depression lasts longer than a few weeks. It affects your daily life and prevents you from doing normal activities. This is long-term depression and should be treated.

Remember, if you are depressed, it's not your fault. You haven't failed. Just as with other health problems, you can get help.

An event can trigger long-term depression, such as the loss of a loved one. But depression can also have physical causes. In some people, chemicals in their body are not in balance. This can cause depression. Changes in hormones can also cause depression. That's why some women get depressed after having a baby.

How do you know if you are depressed? Look at this list of signs:

- You have trouble sleeping that lasts for weeks or months. Or you sleep more than normal and have trouble getting out of bed.
- Your eating habits have changed. You eat much more or much less than normal.
- You feel tired all the time.
- You feel as if you have lost control of your life.
- You have problems dealing with other people.
- You do not "feel like yourself."
- You feel hopeless, confused, or frustrated.
- You don't enjoy things you used to, such as sex, food, or being with friends.
- You feel afraid for no reason.
- You drink a lot of alcohol or take drugs.
- You think about killing yourself.

If you're considering killing yourself, you need help right away. Don't delay. Talk to someone you trust—a doctor, friend, or clergy member. You can also call a crisis hotline.

Do any of these signs apply to you? Have they lasted for more than a few weeks? If so, you may be depressed. If you think you are depressed, you can get help.

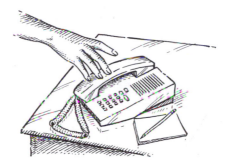

Treatment

If you are depressed, talking about your problem can help. There are trained people who can help you:

- health care provider
- member of the clergy
- social worker
- psychologist
- psychiatrist
- therapist

These people may be able to treat your depression. Or they may refer you to someone else for help.

If the cause of your depression is physical, your doctor may prescribe antidepressants. These are drugs that can ease depression.

There are a few types of antidepressants. They all have side effects. Ask your doctor about the side effects. Decide which ones you can deal with.

Going to the hospital

Some people become so depressed they need constant treatment. They may be a threat to themselves or others. They may not be able to cope at all. When this happens, they may go in the hospital for longer-term care and treatment.

Chapter 6
Sexual Health

Sex is part of being human. It is important to take care of your sexual health. Sexual health includes mental and physical aspects. This chapter covers a range of topics that relate to women's sexual health.

Sexual Parts

The outer sex organs

The vulva is the sex organs on the outside of the body. Two sets of lips surround the openings to the vagina and the urethra (the canal that takes urine from the bladder).

The inner lips join at the front of the body to form the hood of the clitoris. The clitoris is a very sensitive organ that fills with blood during sex. Touching the clitoris can arouse a woman.

The inner sex organs

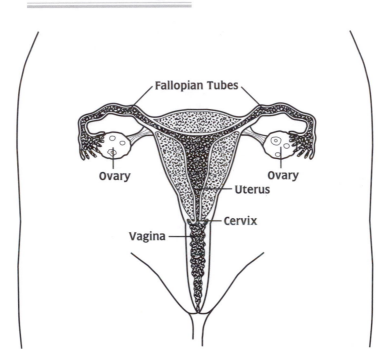

The vagina is the passage that connects the vulva with the uterus (womb). The vagina is made of muscle that changes shape during sex and childbirth. The walls of the vagina produce fluids. These keep the vagina clean and moist.

The uterus is also made of muscle. In a non-pregnant woman, it is the size and shape of a pear. The fetus grows in the uterus during pregnancy. The opening of the uterus is called the cervix.

Two fallopian tubes connect the ovaries to the uterus. Each month, one ovary produces an egg. It travels through the fallopian tube to the uterus.

Breasts

The breasts provide food for a baby. Each breast contains milk glands. When a woman is pregnant, these glands grow to prepare for breast-feeding.

Breasts are also sexual organs. The nipples respond to touch by becoming erect. They also become erect during breast-feeding. This makes it easier for a baby to nurse.

The Menstrual Cycle

The menstrual cycle has about 28 days. The cycle can be shorter or longer, from 23 to 35 days. In healthy women these cycles happen every month until menopause. (Menopause is described in Chapter 7, page 76.) Pregnant women do not have menstrual cycles. Breast-feeding may also stop your menstrual cycle for a time.

Every month or so, a woman's body prepares to get pregnant by releasing an egg. This egg is ready to be fertilized by a sperm.

If the egg is not fertilized, the lining of the uterus breaks down. This lining makes up the menstrual fluid. This part of the cycle is when you have your period.

PMS

Most women get signs that tell them their period is coming. When these become severe, a woman has PMS (premenstrual syndrome). Signs of PMS are depression, mood swings, anger, crying, and confusion. Physical signs are bloating, feeling tired, headache, and swollen breasts. PMS happens just before your period and usually stops when your period starts.

To relieve PMS, try these ideas:

- Avoid caffeine, salt, sugar, and alcohol.
- Eat more starches.
- Try taking calcium, magnesium, and vitamins B6 and E.
- Use the ways to relax on page 51.
- Get regular exercise.

You can also talk to your care provider about treating PMS.

Endometriosis

The tissue that lines the uterus can sometimes grow outside the uterus. When it does, scar tissue can form. These areas can become inflamed and painful. This condition is called endometriosis.

Women with endometriosis usually have bad pain during their periods. They may also feel tired and have diarrhea. Some cannot get pregnant. If you have these signs, see your care provider. It could be endometriosis or something else a doctor should treat.

Sexual Orientation

Most women are attracted to men and choose male partners. They are heterosexual.

About one in every 10 women is attracted to other women. They may choose women as partners. These women are lesbian.

Other women feel attracted to both men and women. They are bisexual. They may have partners of either sex.

Being heterosexual, lesbian, or bisexual is a person's sexual orientation. People don't choose their sexual orientation—it just is.

Lesbians and health care

Lesbians need to have the routine exams described in Chapter 4, page 33. This is true even if they don't plan to have children. Some lesbians feel uncomfortable with health care providers. A woman may not want to reveal she is lesbian. She may not want to answer questions about birth control. If you are a lesbian, try to find a health care provider whom you trust.

Women can get STDs (sexually transmitted diseases), including AIDS, from other women. Lesbians need to know their sexual partners' histories and protect themselves, just as women who have sex with men do.

Masturbation

Masturbation means touching yourself for sexual pleasure. This is normal and OK. Men, women, gays, lesbians, and heterosexuals all do it. Masturbating won't cause health problems.

Masturbating can help you understand your own body. It can help your sexual relationship with a partner.

Problems with Sex

Most people have problems with sex at some point. Some of these problems are

- little or no desire for sex
- not feeling aroused
- not having orgasms
- painful sex

Emotional problems

Problems with sex most often have to do with your feelings. They may result from problems you are having with your partner, or from bad sexual experiences in the past.

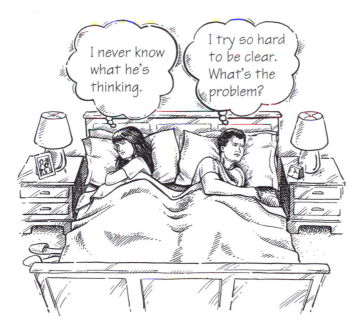

If you are having problems with sex, try to talk with your partner. Being honest about how you feel is the first step to overcoming your problems.

Talking to other women may help, too. You may find that they have the same concerns and fears as you do. They may have ideas that can help.

Some problems with sex are too hard to solve alone. Your care provider can help you find a counselor or a therapist.

Physical problems

Some problems with sex are physical. Painful sex is often the result of an infection or endometriosis. If sex is often painful for you, see your care provider. He may be able to prescribe treatment or exercises that will help.

Vaginal Infections

Most women will get a vaginal infection, or vaginitis, at some point in their lives.

There is always some discharge from the vagina. This discharge helps keep the vagina clean. A change in this discharge can signal an infection. The signs of vaginitis are

- burning or itching around the vagina
- more discharge than normal

- a colored discharge (could be white, cream colored, yellow, yellow-green, or gray)
- discharge that has an odor (could be foul-smelling, fishy, or yeasty)
- pain during sex
- pain during urination

If you have any of these symptoms, check with your care provider. She can decide what kind of treatment you need. In some cases, your sex partner may need treatment too.

Birth control pills make women more likely to get vaginal infections. Some women have to stop taking the birth control pills to clear up the infection.

Preventing vaginal infections

Here are some ways to prevent getting vaginal infections:

- Avoid tight clothes that can keep the vaginal area moist and warm.
- Wash the vaginal area every day.
- Wear clean cotton underpants. This helps keep the vaginal area dry.
- Don't use perfumed soaps or vaginal sprays.
- Use undyed (white) toilet paper.
- After going to the bathroom, wipe from

front to back. This keeps germs away from your vagina.

- Don't douche. Your vagina keeps itself clean.

- If your vagina is dry, don't have sex. Or use a water-based lubricant during sex.

Sexually Transmitted Diseases (STDs)

Sexually transmitted diseases (called STDs) are passed from person to person during sex. You cannot get an STD from toilet seats or other objects. Some common STDs are gonorrhea, genital warts, herpes, syphilis, and chlamydia.

AIDS can be spread by sex, too. See page 69 for information on women and AIDS.

Most STDs can be treated and cured. But it is best not to get an STD in the first place. The only way to be sure not to get an STD is not to have sex. If you do have sex, follow these safer sex tips to avoid getting an STD.

- If your partner is a man, use latex condoms. Make sure your partner puts on the condom before his penis touches you.

- During oral sex, use some form of protection (a dental dam, plastic wrap, or a non-lubricated condom that you have cut open). Make sure that there is no contact between the mouth and the sex parts.

- Don't have many sex partners. The fewer partners you have, the less chance you have of getting an STD.
- Ask any sex partners about their sex history. By having sex with a person, you are exposed to any germs that person got from another partner.

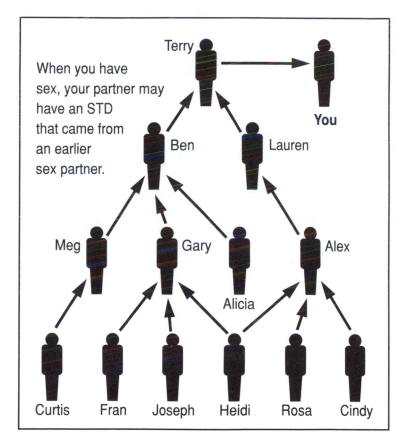

When you have sex, your partner may have an STD that came from an earlier sex partner.

Terry

You

Ben   Lauren

Meg   Gary   Alex

Alicia

Curtis   Fran   Joseph   Heidi   Rosa   Cindy

If you get an STD

If you think you may have an STD, go to your health care provider right away. He can test you for STDs and start treatment.

If you do have an STD, your sex partners should be tested and treated too.

If your doctor prescribes antibiotics as treatment, it's best not to have sex. You can still spread the STD then. If you do have sex, use latex condoms. If you take birth control pills, they may not work while you take antibiotics. That's another reason to use a condom.

Pelvic Inflammatory Disease (PID)

About 1 million women in the U.S. get pelvic inflammatory disease (PID) each year. PID is a serious STD. It usually starts as a simple STD. If that infection is not treated, it can spread and become PID.

Signs of PID

- pain in the belly
- unusual discharge from vagina
- fever or chills
- feeling like you have the flu
- bleeding after sex

- painful sex
- dizziness
- bleeding between periods
- pain when you pass urine
- back or leg pain

If you think you might have PID, go to your care provider. If you do have PID, your treatment should start soon. You'll have a better chance of being cured.

Women and AIDS

AIDS is caused by a virus called HIV. HIV lives in the blood, sex fluids, and breast milk of an infected person.

HIV can be passed from one person to another through sex and through sharing needles for IV drug use. A pregnant woman can also pass HIV to her unborn baby.

Here are some facts about HIV/AIDS:

- HIV is spreading fastest in the U.S. among women, teenagers, African Americans, and Latinos.
- Women are more likely than men to get HIV through heterosexual sex.
- Rough sex and anal sex increase the risk of passing the virus.

- A pregnant woman with HIV who gets treatment reduces the chance of passing HIV to her baby to 1 in 10. If she is not treated, it rises to 3 or 4 in 10. If you are pregnant and could have been exposed to HIV, get tested. A simple blood test may save your baby.
- If you have sex, only latex condoms can protect you from HIV. Lambskin condoms and other forms of birth control can't.

HIV cannot be passed by casual contact.

Casual Contact - Safe	
touching	shaking hands
hugging	sneezing
coughing	kissing on the cheek
toilet seats	bathtubs
swimming pools	water fountains
glasses or cups	dishes
telephones	office equipment
pens	furniture (chairs, beds, etc.)
towels	clothing
exercise equipment	mosquitoes or other insects
animals	giving blood
knives, forks, or spoons	food prepared by an HIV+ person

Women need to protect themselves from getting HIV. Not having intercourse at all is the surest way to prevent getting HIV/AIDS from sex. If you do have sex, you should practice safer sex. Safer sex reduces the risk of passing or getting HIV.

Safer sex

The main rule for safer sex is: don't let someone else's body fluids inside your body. Latex condoms are the best way to reduce your risk of getting HIV/AIDS or any STD. You can buy them at any drugstore.

Choose condoms with these words on the package: *latex, disease prevention, water-based lubricant,* and *spermicide* or *nonoxynol-9*.

You can also use a condom that fits inside a woman, but it may not protect you as well against STDs and HIV.

Birth Control

Birth control lets you decide whether or not you want to get pregnant. There are many birth control methods. Most are very safe. Some are more effective than others. The chart on pages 72–73 lists some common types.

Barrier Methods		
Cervical Cap	**Condom**	**Diaphragm**
When you use this method ➡ Your doctor fits you with a thimble-shaped latex cap. You coat it with spermicide and put it in your vagina before intercourse.	➡ You put the condom on the erect penis before intercourse. (Note: Condoms are most effective when used with spermicides.)	➡ Your doctor fits you with a shallow latex cap. You coat it with spermicide and put it in your vagina before intercourse.
Effectiveness ➡ 82% – 94%	➡ 88% – 98%	➡ 82% – 94%
Pros ➡ can last for several years ➡ comfortable and cheap	➡ easy and cheap to buy	➡ can last for several years
Cons ➡ can be messy ➡ can't be used during bleeding or infection ➡ can be difficult to fit and to use	➡ can break ➡ can reduce feeling	➡ can be messy ➡ can't be used during bleeding or infection ➡ increases risk of bladder infection

Hormone Methods		
Depo-Provera	**Norplant**	**The Pill**
When you use this method ➡ Your doctor gives you a hormone shot every 12 weeks.	➡ Your doctor puts six small capsules in your arm.	➡ You take one pill once a day.
Effectiveness ➡ 99.7%	➡ 99.96%	➡ 97% – 99.9%
Pros ➡ nothing to put in place before intercourse	➡ lasts for five years ➡ nothing to remember ➡ can be removed any time	➡ nothing to put in place before intercourse ➡ more regular periods ➡ less cramping, acne, anemia, and PMS
Cons ➡ side effects, including irregular bleeding, weight gain, headaches, depression, and stomach pain ➡ side effects last until shot wears off ➡ may cause delay in getting pregnant after shots are stopped	➡ requires minor surgery ➡ side effects, including irregular bleeding, headaches, depression, and weight gain	➡ must be taken daily ➡ rare but serious health risks ➡ side effects, including temporary irregular bleeding

| Other Methods | | | |
Abstinence	IUD	Natural Family Planning	Sterilization
When you use this method ➡ You don't have vaginal intercourse.	➡ Your doctor puts a small plastic device inside your uterus.	➡ You chart your cycle and use physical signs to predict fertile days. On those days, you don't have intercourse, or you use a barrier method.	➡ You have surgery to block your fallopian tubes.
Effectiveness ➡ 100%	➡ 97.4% – 99.2%	➡ 80% – 99%	➡ 99.6% – 99.8%
Pros ➡ no side effects ➡ no cost	➡ nothing to put in place before intercourse	➡ no side effects ➡ supplies (calendars, thermometers, charts) cheap and easy to get	➡ permanent ➡ nothing to remember ➡ no lasting side effects
Cons ➡ difficult for many people	➡ can cause cramps, spotting between periods, longer and heavier periods ➡ can cause infection and sterility	➡ requires careful record-keeping ➡ abstaining on fertile days can be difficult ➡ not effective if your cycle is irregular	➡ cannot be reversed ➡ requires surgery ➡ can fail in rare cases

How birth control works

For a woman to get pregnant, her egg must join with a man's sperm. This is called fertilization. Most forms of birth control prevent the egg and sperm from joining.

There are two main types of birth control.

- Hormone methods prevent your body from releasing an egg.
- Barrier methods keep your egg and your partner's sperm apart. They are often used with a spermicide, which kills sperm.

Other types of birth control are IUDs, sterilization, and natural methods (including abstinence).

You and your partner can discuss which birth control method is best for you. Talk with your health care provider too.

If you take birth control pills, they may not work while you take antibiotics. Be sure to use condoms for backup.

Unwanted Pregnancy

No birth control method (except abstinence) is 100 percent effective. Even sterilization can fail. You may become pregnant when you don't want to. If this happens you have choices. What you decide to do is very personal, but talking to doctors and other people can help.

You may decide to go ahead with the pregnancy and keep the child. You may decide to have the child and place it for adoption. Or you may decide to have an abortion.

This is your decision. Don't let anyone— your partner, parents, or a care provider— pressure you. Take into account your situation and your own values and beliefs.

Abortion is a way of ending a pregnancy. Abortions are safest in the early stages of pregnancy. If you think you may want to have an abortion, talk to your care provider or go to a women's health clinic. Talk to someone you trust, and do what's best for you.

There is no proof that having one abortion affects your being able to have children later on. But repeat abortions may have serious effects.

Chapter 7

As Women Get Older

Truths about Getting Older

- Even though older women can't give birth, they still need to see a care provider regularly.
- Healthy eating and exercise are just as important as you get older.
- Many older women have active sex lives.

Many women live a healthy, happy life well into their 80s and beyond. But you must take care of yourself. You need to be aware of the changing needs of your body.

Medical Tests

As you age, your risk of getting certain diseases increases. It's important to see your care provider regularly. After you reach 65, your care provider may want to do more tests. The tests can find disease early and help you live longer. Common tests for older women are

- Pap test
- mammogram
- test for low iron
- cholesterol screening

You and your care provider will decide how often to do the tests. How often depends partly on your medical history.

Food and Exercise

Healthy eating and exercise are part of staying well for everyone. However, your needs change as you get older.

Healthy eating

After menopause, women are more likely to get osteoporosis. Osteoporosis weakens bones and may cause fractures. Women with this condition may have curved backs. To prevent it, you need calcium and exercise. Experts recommend that after menopause women get 1,500 milligrams of calcium a day. Look on page 13 for some good sources of calcium. Most older women need calcium supplements, too.

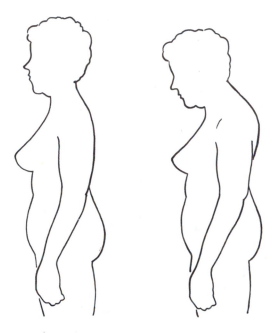

Many older women get constipated. They may need to eat more fiber to prevent constipation. Fiber helps remove waste from the body. Fruits, vegetables, and grains are high in fiber.

Your eating habits may change as you get older. You may eat less. You may eat the same but notice that you are gaining weight. Any extreme weight gain or loss may be a problem. You should check with your care provider about it.

Exercise

Older women who follow an exercise program enjoy better health. Regular exercise can reduce your risk of

- heart disease
- high blood pressure
- diabetes
- osteoporosis
- obesity

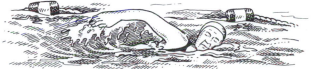

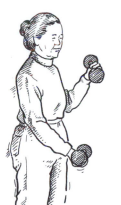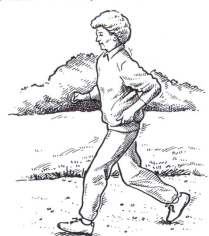

Exercise also helps reduce

- shortness of breath
- sleeplessness
- loss of bone
- back pain and stiffness
- weak muscles
- depression

If you have not been exercising, talk with your care provider before you begin. She can help you choose the types of exercise that are right for you. Start slowly and avoid exercises that can jar your body. Some good activities for older women include

- walking
- swimming
- light weight lifting
- low-impact aerobics

Heart Disease and Stroke

As you get older, your risk of heart disease and stroke increases. Heart disease kills more women in the U.S. than any other disease. Here are five key ways to have a healthy heart.

Quit smoking. Quitting smoking is the best thing you can do to reduce your risk of heart disease. Women who smoke are six times as likely as nonsmokers to have a heart attack. Chapter 3 has information on quitting smoking.

Control your high blood pressure. Some people can control high blood pressure by losing weight, changing their diet, and cutting down on sodium. Other people need to take drugs to control it. Talk to your care provider about what you can do.

Reduce blood cholesterol. Your care provider can measure the amount of cholesterol in your blood. When cholesterol builds up in your blood, it can cause heart disease. If your cholesterol is high, you may need to lose weight, change your eating habits, or both. Talk to your care provider about what you can do.

Control your weight. If you are overweight, talk to your care provider. Together, you can develop a plan for losing weight safely.

Control stress in your life. Too much stress can increase your risk of heart disease. See Chapter 5 for ideas for reducing stress.

Menopause

Menopause is the time of life when you stop having your period. You cannot become pregnant naturally after menopause. Most women go through menopause at around age 50, but it can happen before or after that age.

Your period will probably not stop all of a sudden. You may skip a period or two. Your period may get lighter. You may have heavy bleeding sometimes. This can happen for three to five years.

Other changes

You may have other changes with menopause. Many women get hot flashes. These are feelings of intense heat in your body. Hot flashes can cause sweating in the day or in the night. They can last for just a moment or up to half an hour.

Here are some tips for dealing with hot flashes:

- Dress in layers. That way, you can remove a layer to get cool.
- Drink a glass of cold water or juice when a hot flash starts.
- Keep ice water by your bed.
- Wear cotton clothes and use cotton sheets.

The skin in your vagina changes as you age. It becomes thinner and dryer. This can make sex uncomfortable. You can use water-based lubricants to help.

Your urinary tract changes too. You may pass urine without wanting to. This can be caused by illness or by coughing, sneezing, laughing, or heavy lifting. In most cases, passing urine this way can be treated. Talk to your care provider.

Mental health

Some women find that menopause and the time after is the best period of their lives. Women in menopause are no more likely to get depressed than younger women.

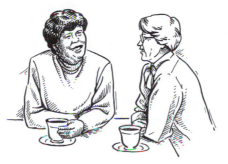

However, women who have had their ovaries removed are more likely to be depressed than other women.

Sometimes older women get depressed because of other changes in their life. Divorce, the death of loved ones, or children leaving home can trigger depression. Pages 55–56 are about treatment for depression.

Treatment

The signs of menopause are caused by a drop in female hormones. Some women find these signs uncomfortable.

Hormone replacement therapy (HRT) can help. HRT provides hormones (estrogen and progesterone) that an older woman's body makes less of. The benefits of HRT are

- relief from hot flashes
- moister tissue in the vagina
- less risk of osteoporosis
- less risk of heart disease

HRT is *not* a good choice for all women. It can cause side effects such as

- bloating
- tender breasts
- mood swings

And studies show that estrogen increases the risk of getting cancer of the uterus. It may also increase the risk of breast cancer. (Adding progesterone may help reduce those added risks.)

For these reasons, HRT is not safe for all women. Look at the following list. If anything on it is true for you, you should probably not take HRT. Talk to your care provider about it.

- Your mother or sister had breast cancer.
- You have high blood pressure.
- You have had a stroke.
- You have liver disease.
- You have diabetes.
- You have varicose veins.
- You get migraine headaches.
- You have gallbladder trouble.
- You have fibroids in your uterus.
- Your mother took the drug DES when she was pregnant.

If HRT is not right for you, you and your care provider can talk about other ways to deal with menopause. Talk with other women to find out what works for them.

Sex

Women can enjoy sex all their lives. About one in three women find they have less sex drive as they age. This may be caused by changing hormone levels. If your vagina becomes dry, you can use lubricants when you have sex. Estrogen creams can help, too. If you are concerned about not enjoying sex, talk to your care provider.

Chapter 8

Violence against Women

Think about these figures:

- More than 2 million women report being abused by their partner each year in the U.S.
- 1 in 8 women in the U.S. has been raped.
- Up to 25 percent of women were sexually abused as children.

The numbers could be even higher. The fact is, women are at risk. Women are less at risk from strangers than from people they know. Most abuse comes from husbands, partners, fathers, and other family members.

Domestic Abuse

Your care provider may ask you if you have ever been beaten. Don't be offended. The American Medical Association tells doctors to check all women patients for signs of domestic violence or abuse. This is because so many women are victims of abuse.

Experts guess that between 30 and 40 percent of emergency room visits by women are the result of domestic violence. Women suffer broken bones, bruises, and damage to all parts of their bodies. Most injuries are on the chest, head, neck, breasts, and belly.

Domestic abuse is a way of gaining control. It is also a crime. A woman can be abused in either a heterosexual or a lesbian relationship. In most cases though, men are the abusers. A man beats his partner to show her that he holds the power. In turn, the abused woman starts to doubt herself. Her self-esteem goes down. She may forget that no one deserves to be beaten. The illustration on page 88 shows the cycle of abuse.

This pattern repeats itself over and over. Each time, the woman thinks less of herself. She becomes more afraid. It becomes harder for her to leave her partner.

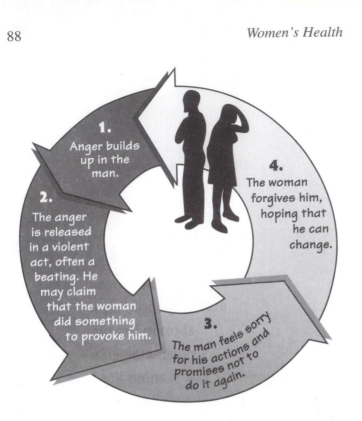

Men who abuse their partners often have things in common. They

- may need to control the world around them
- may have been raised in a violent home
- may abuse alcohol or drugs
- may be jealous of their partners

Leaving

Most experts say you should leave a dangerous partner. However, leaving an abuser is hard. Many abused women are afraid that their partner will kill them if they try to leave. And some abusers do kill.

Money can also be a problem. If the woman has little or no income, she may fear she can't support herself and her children.

But you can get help if you are being abused. Family and friends can be a good source of support. A local women's shelter can also help. Look in the phone book or call the numbers on page 94 for help.

You may want to make a plan for leaving. Here are some tips for preparing:

- Plan where you will go when you leave. A shelter and the home of friends or family are some choices. You may want a place your partner doesn't know about.
- Save enough money to get there. If you can, put money aside to live on for a short time, too. (But if you don't have money, don't wait to save it.)
- Keep a record of the abuse. If you can, take photos of your injuries. Keep police reports.

The list on page 90 shows how a woman might get ready to leave an abusive partner. The list includes things that are good for a woman to take when she leaves. She checks off items she has. She crosses out items that don't apply to her. She makes notes on a few items.

Things to Take When You Leave

Identification
- ✓ Social Security cards
- ✓ driver's license
- ~~welfare identification~~
- ✓ birth certificates for self and children
- ~~passports, green cards,~~
  ~~work permits~~

Financial
- ✓ money
- ~~bankbook~~
- ✓ checkbook
- ✓ credit cards
- ~~mortgage payment book~~
- ✓ current unpaid bills
- insurance papers *can't find*

Other legal papers
- ✓ car registration
- ~~divorce papers~~
- lease or ~~house deed~~ *can't find*

Personal
- ✓ keys to house, car, ~~& office~~
- ~~medications~~
- ✓ change of clothes
- ✓ pictures, jewelry, items of sentimental value
- ✓ children's favorite toys or blankets

Important records
- ✓ school records
- ✓ address book
- medical records *at doctor's office*

But if you or your children are in danger, don't wait to collect these things. Leave when you need to.

Rape

Rape is forced sex. In many states, this means any kind of sexual contact without both partners agreeing. Almost all rapists are men.

Men who rape do it in order to have power over their victim. They want to make her feel shame. They do not rape for sexual pleasure. Rape is not about sex; it's violence.

In four out of five rapes, the woman knows the man. He may be a date, her husband, or a family member. It's not true that most rapes are done by strangers.

It's also not true that women "ask" to be raped. Rape is never the victim's fault.

Preventing rape

There is no way to keep yourself completely safe from rape. But you can take steps to make rape less likely. Here are some ideas:

- Avoid drinking too much alcohol or taking drugs.
- Firmly tell any date to stop if he pressures you to have sex.
- Don't go home with a man you just met.
- Consider taking a course in self-defense for women.

These ideas may help prevent an attack by a stranger:

- Don't walk alone at night.
- Always keep your home and car locked.

- Don't hitchhike or get into cars with strangers.
- Use only your first initial on your mailbox and in the phone book.

If you are raped

If you are raped, you need medical care right away. You may need to go to a hospital emergency room. Don't bathe or take a shower first. You will wash away proof of the rape.

Many towns and cities have rape hotlines or rape crisis centers you can call. They can help you decide what to do and offer you support.

Rape hotlines can also help if you were raped a long time ago. The counselors can talk with you about your feelings. They may also be able to tell you about local support groups. Many women find such groups helpful.

Child Sex Abuse

Some experts think that up to one in every four women were victims of sex abuse as children. Most of this abuse is done by fathers, stepfathers, and other family members.

Sex abuse of children is

- using sexual language that makes children feel bad or scares them
- oral sex

- vaginal sex
- anal sex
- any kind of sexual contact

Child sex abuse affects a victim's whole life. Many people push away the memories and don't remember being abused. But the effects are still there. They may have trouble trusting others. They may not be able to form lasting bonds with other people.

If you were a victim of sex abuse as a child, you need to get help. Counseling can help you understand how the abuse has affected you. Your care provider can suggest a therapist to help you. There are also support groups in many communities.

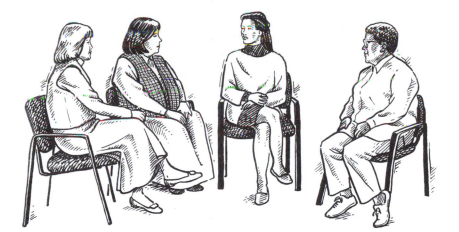

Resources

General

National Women's Health Network
(202) 347-1140
Ask for the number of the group nearest you.

The Women's Complete Health Book
This book, from the American Medical Women's Association, gives more detailed information on women's health. You can buy it in bookstores.

Violence against Women

National Domestic Violence Hotline
(800) 799-SAFE (7233)

National Coalition against Domestic Violence
(303) 839-1852

Smoking, Alcohol, and Drugs

American Cancer Society
Look in the phone book for your local chapter.

The Cancer Information Service
(800) 4-CANCER (422-6237)

National Clearinghouse for Alcohol and Drug Information

> (800) 729-6686

National Drug Information Treatment and Referral Line

> (800) 662-HELP (662-4357)—English
> (800) 66-AYUDA (662-9832)—Spanish

Alcoholics Anonymous

> (212) 870-3400

Women for Sobriety

> (215) 536-8026

Narcotics Anonymous

> (818) 780-3951

Sexual Health

Planned Parenthood

> Look in the phone book for your local chapter.

National Women's Health Network

> (202) 347-1140

Breast Care and Cancer Support

National Alliance of Breast Cancer Organizations

> (800) 719-9154

Susan G. Komen Breast Cancer Foundation

> (800) 462-9273

Y-Me

> (800) 221-2141

Nutrition

The American Dietetic Association
(800) 366-1655

Exercise

American Heart Association
Look in the phone book for your local office.

Women's Sports Foundation
(800) 227-3988

YWCA
Look in the phone book for your local YWCA.

Women and Aging

National Osteoporosis Foundation
(202) 223-2226

National Institute on Aging
(800) 222-2225

Older Women's League
(800) TAKE-OWL (825-3695)

Mental Health Matters

DEPRESSION Awareness, Recognition, and Treatment Program
National Institute of Mental Health
(301) 421-4211

National Mental Health Association (NMHA)
(800) 969-6642